POETRY

SIT WITH ME
ANOTHER WHILE LONGER
The Collected Works of
Michael A. Horvich
2013-2021

POETRY

SIT WITH ME
ANOTHER WHILE LONGER
The Collected Works of
Michael A. Horvich
2013-2021

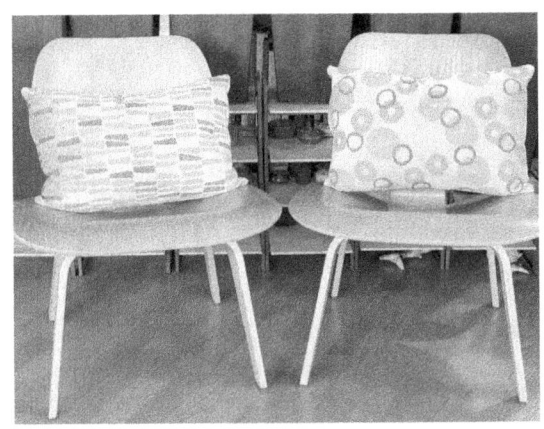

Ragdale Foundation - Ring Gala
Lake Forest, Il - 2013

First Printing: 2014

ISBN 978-1-329-81901-6

Michael A. Horvich
807 Davis St Suite 415
Evanston, Illinois 60201

www.horvich.com
m@horvich.com

ACKNOWLEDGEMENTS

How does one go about thanking all those to whom thanks are due?

Apologize ahead of time to those you will forget to mention?

Arrange the names in alphabetical order so as not to have to prioritize the importance of any one individual? Worse, try to rank them in some particular order?

Begin with thanking ones parents, to whom you owe your very being? Thank your loving family?

Thank your life partner and spiritual mate for not only putting up with you but also supporting you and helping to foster your growth over all these years?

Thank your pets, living and deceased, who have always given you unqualified love and joy?

Daunting job. So on the next page, let me quote instead from a poem I came across ... and add a few words of my own:

TENDERLY

Tenderly, I now touch all things,

Knowing one day we will part.

St. John of the Cross, born Juan de Yepes y Alvarez, 1542-91

THANK YOU

To everyone who has touched me and who

hopefully I have touched in return. Sit with me a

while longer yet!

DEDICATION

The expression "Until Death Do you Part" in the marriage ceremony is erroneous! Gregory died peacefully in 2015 having lived well with Dementia/Alzheimer's Disease for 12 years.

Although he died six years ago, our love is as strong as ever and it continues to grow in new ways, even though he is no longer physically available to me.

The grief never ends, it just changes. I continue to grow so the grief becomes easier to carry.

I miss him every day, I talk to him every day, I see him in my mind's eye every day. I will carry my grief until the end of my days.

Great love brings great grief! I wouldn't have it any other way!

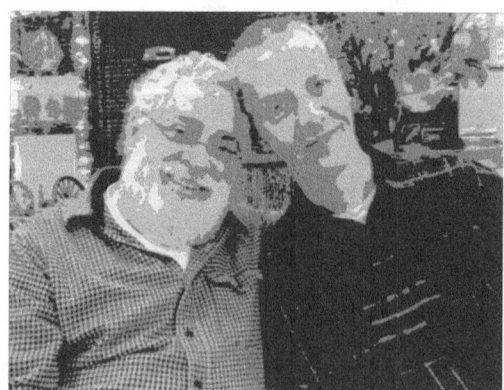

Michael & Gregory
Evanston, IL – 2013

POETRY

SIT WITH ME
ANOTHER WHILE LONGER
The Collected Works of
Michael A. Horvich
2013-2021

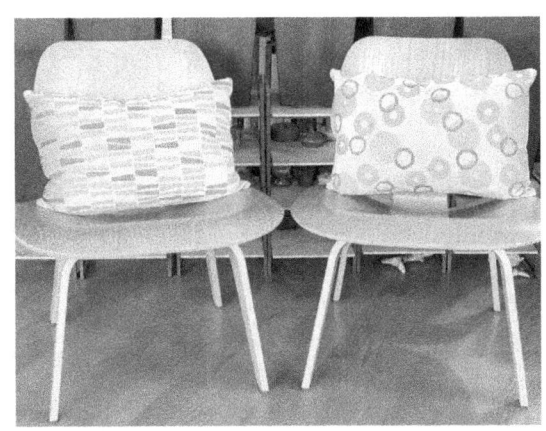

TABLE OF CONTENTS

POETRY

AN
INTRODUCTION

✳ ✳ ✳

SECTION ONE

<u>Writing Corner</u>

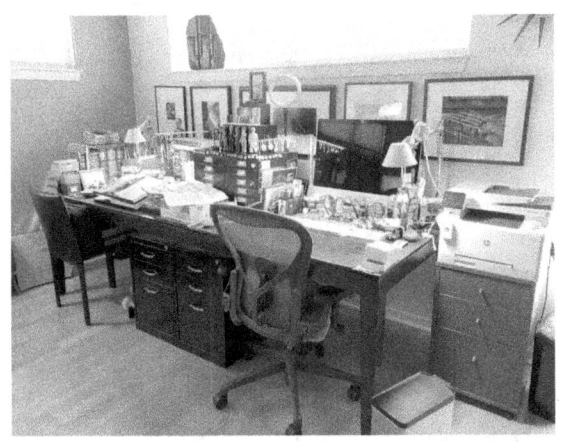

My writing space is in the living room of my condo in Evanston, Illinois. Based on the sage advice of many writers, "Write every day, even if you have nothing to say!" I sit here, in front of my computer, several hours a day thinking, writing, editing, formatting, and finally publishing my works. See APPENDIX for a list of my other publications.

Introduction

I find writing helps me process, understand, problem solve, and figure out my life. Some times that writing takes the form of poetry. I am not the first to say this, but at times it is as if poetry choses me, I do not choose it.

What I find in poetry is beauty, hope, clarity, faith, and life. Poetry deals with the essence. The words are carefully chosen, the images carefully drawn, the ideas carefully woven.

Much of my poetry was informed by Gregory's diagnosis of and living with Dementia/ Alzheimer's.

As his communication abilities and cognitive skills diminished, he was not available to me in the sharing of our day-to-day joys and sorrows.

Writing, for me, therefore became an important way of supporting myself emotionally and intellectually and giving myself closure to difficult moments where real closure was not available.

My poetry slowed down as my life became calmer and the crisis of Dementia/Alzheimer's passed with Gregory's death, but my writing continues to be an important part of my everyday life.

POETRY
WHILE ON THE ALZHEIMER'S PATH

✳ ✳ ✳

SECTION TWO

<u>Always - 07/04/13</u>

I will always love Gregory

I do not want to be afraid.

I do not want to be angry.

I do not want to be sad.

I only want to be kind.

I only want to be loving.

I only want to be understanding.

I only want to be supportive.

I am working on changing.

I have changed my "DO NOT WANTS"

And changed my "ONLY WANTS"

To "I AM's"

I am always going to love Gregory.

I am not afraid.

I am not angry.

I am not sad.

I am kind.

I am loving.

I am understanding.

I am supportive.

✳ ✳ ✳

How Does It Feel – 07/22/13

Like a switch being turned off

Like a fog rolling in

A numbness overtakes me

I stare into the distance.

An emptiness that feels like sorrow

A pain that feels like an ache

A sadness overtakes me

I stare into the abyss.

Without an understanding

Of what really happened

Or a way of explaining

What actually went wrong.

And then the clouds disappear

And life reenters the picture

With dishes to be done

And laundry to be folded.

The Exchange – 01/31/15

"I don't want to stay, to stay.

I want to see, to see, to see."

A brief flicker of sadness in him

Then his notice of sadness in me

Followed by his apology:

"I am sorry. I am sorry."

Then my giving permission:

"Say what you have to."

"Really?"

"Yes."

✳ ✳ ✳

Crying Myself - 02/21/15

Crying Myself Silently

Without making a squeak or loud noises

I have learned to cry myself silently

But tears still as large as sobs

A song, an idea, a line in a play

Bring on a wave of emotions

I have learned to cry myself silently

But tears still as large as rivers

A thought, a memory, a photograph

Bring on an attack of emotions

I have learned to cry myself silently

But tears still as oceans

Over time, I have learned to say

Thank you emotions

Thank you tears

Just not right now

I have learned to cry silently.

✳ ✳ ✳

Yesterday at Lieberman – 02/24/15

"I love you very much."

No notice.

"I love you more than the highest mountain."

Head turned towards me but **no** focus.

"I love you more than the deepest ocean."

Head turned towards me **with** focus.

"I love you more than all the stars in the sky."

Looking at me with a quivering chin.

"I love you more than all the desert sand."

One tear rolls down his cheek.

"Why?" he says.

"Because you are wonderful."

"You are handsome, intelligent. and kind."

More tears roll down his cheek.

"I will always love you, be here for you."

Time to hug him, and rock, and cry with him.

✳ ✳ ✳

Boink Love – 03/01/15

Gregory sitting in his wheelchair

Me sitting next to him on a stool

He leans in towards me

I lean in towards him

He leans in closer to me

I lean in closer yet to him

Our foreheads touch

"Boink," he says.

How It Is Now – 06/07/15

The key in the door turns

The memories are silent

Hiding least they evoke

Difficult memories.

Over the threshold one steps

Into the waiting abyss

The house filled to overflowing

With every last encounter.

Into the front hall closet

Onto the waiting hanger

You place your jacket gingerly

With others no longer owned.

Walking past the lonely bedroom

Into the front of the condo

Shelved and collected and scattered

With mementos, memorabilia, reminders.

Two grocery bags filled

With individual items

Then emptied into the cabinets

And refrigerator ... for one.

Dinner from the microwave
Emptied on a tray and taken
Into the TV room TV table
For flickering eating friendships.

The cats, two of them purring
Bringing life and joy to you
Without expectations to be filled
Joy on the shoulders of sorrow.

Then bedtime with the wrinkled sheets
Only your scent and your pillows
And the memories no longer silent
Keeping the night long and loving.

These Leavings – 06/15/15

One spends time visiting
In his new space
Me, the only one
Who really knows
Really Understands.

And then comes time
For me to leave him
Returning to my home
So I cry and grieve
Yet another leaving.

And my condo
Is once again filled
To overflowing
With emptiness
Being alone.

The reality of it
Needing to be cried
But rarely allowed
Announces and arrives
In torrents.

"I knooooooo ... I knooooooo," I wail to myself.
With tears pouring out, but I don't really know.
Afraid to lose myself in the river of grief,
Unable to breath, afraid of getting lost in side.
"I knooooooo," I wail.

And then another day
Of getting through life.
Finding joy here and there,
A laugh or two or three,
Always on shoulders of sorrow.

❋ ❋ ❋

<u>Windows – 06/25/15</u>

Imagining the Windows of Gregory's Mind.

What must they see?

At what must they look out?

What do they see

When they look in?

Does the sun shine brightly

With flowers in bloom

And birds hopping from tree to tree?

Leaves fluttering in the breeze

And the soft smell of Spring in the air?

Or is the day overcast?

Flowers nowhere to be seen

No sound to disturb one's lacks

Nonsense flickering on the TV screen

And the scent of lavender room spray?

✳ ✳ ✳

<u>Reminders – 06/30/15</u>

Tears

Are a constant

Which help to remind us

That we are alive.

Joy,

Even though carried

On the shoulders of Sorrow,

Also reminds us of this.

<u>Memories – 07/28/15</u>

Memories of earlier times arrive
No longer to be there for me, or us
So I sit at computer and compose
And console self as best I can.

I sit on the summer warmed balcony
The grass and trees growing lush
On the roof deck garden below us
As this poem begins to blur.

My coffee steams in the hot sun
My toast: rye with raspberry jam
The birds chirp and tweet and twittle
As the cold tears wet my cheeks.

"May I come out and join you?" he asks
With an up turned questioning voice
"But off course you may and welcome!"
As I reply with sorrow's memory.

We talk about flowers below us growing
About the sun and clouds above us moving
We sit together quietly holding hands
As my memory is unable to quiet itself.

I stick my expecting bare feet into
His empty, sun warmed worn sandals
He suns his legs stretched over mine
And I wonder with whom can I cry?

Deep gasp after gasp after breath
Tears continuing to flood and fill
A sadness, an emptiness, a grief
So deep as to drown without hope.

Medically Speaking – 08/17/15

Every now and then when least expected

The wound that is Dementia/Alzheimer's

Reopens and I bleed again a little more.

It will probably never heal completely

And I do not expect or hope for it to do so

The pain does become a little more bearable

The reality of it and the implications hit

When I lease expect it and I have no one

With whom to cry, so I sob and sob and howl

The one person who used to help me cope

Is inadvertently the one person who now

Is the reason for the emotions, the sorrow

He is still able to help but in a different way

In a very different capacity so now I must

In most ways be strong for him and for me

I am quickly able to staunch the flow of pain

Go back to experiencing and acknowledging

Life's joy carried on sorrow's shoulders.

✳ ✳ ✳

Connections – 08/26/15

These moments are precious
They will be remembered forever
As he looked into my eyes.

He smiled and
He said, "I love you."
I melted and said, "I love you too."

This was yesterday
Coming from somewhere deep within
Bubbling forth from Gregory.

"I love you." to let me know
He is with me still
Different and the same.

Somehow his body
And his spirit connected
And the best of him shined forth.

And our love reached new heights.
I love that man.
"More Than Ever!"

* * *

A Trip to The Barber – 09/04/15

Gregory lifted his arm slowly

And with finger stiffly aimed,

He pointed at my beard.

"Yes," I replied

As if I knew what he would say,

"I had my beard trimmed."

I also got my hair cut.

See how short it is!"

I leaned in towards him.

He lifted his arm slowly

And navigating thoughtfully,

He ruffled the hair on my head.

This unexpected interaction

Between us spontaneously,

Rekindled the human connection.

I loved the feel of his tender touch.

He loved the feel of touching me.

Another Monumental Momentary Miracle!

✳ ✳ ✳

*Gregory passed on
October 4, 2015*

Gregory's Passing – 10/18/15

Gregory died on October 4, 2015

Which was only two weeks ago

An eternity of Sundays

It seems like forever

It seems like yesterday

It seems like soon to come.

Forty years together

Just a day has passed

A lifetime continues

How long is a moment?

How long is a lifetime

How long is love

Forever and a day

Yet to come?

Or a lifetime continuing.

✳ ✳ ✳

A Life So Quickly – 10/19/15

What is a life?

A moment in the day?

A memory to think of?

The passage of time?

Why does it go so quickly?

Where does it go in the end?

What is a life?

Living to the fullest.

Family and Friends.

Lovers and loved ones.

Why does it go so quickly?

Where does it go in the end?

What is a life?

A photograph, a video.

A love letter with flowers.

A special gift to cherish.

Why does it go so quickly?

Where does it go in the end?

What is a life?

A kiss hello and one goodbye.

That special smile and wink.

A hug that doesn't stop.

Why does it go so quickly?

Where does it go in the end?

Slow down! Don't miss it!

Where does it go in the end?

You carry it in your heart.

What is a life?

Ménage À Trois - Written 06/15/12

35 years and their relationship is as strong as ever.

Love continuing to grow, change, adjust.

Uninvited, a third partner joined the relationship.

It was not fashionable when they first fell in love,

Unacceptable for two of the same sex to do so.

Let alone a third participant in a relationship.

But Alzheimer's does not discriminate.

Dementia does not ask permission.

So it became a ménage à trois.

Each one was very much unlike the other.

He was tall, fair, and thoughtful.

He was short, dark, and enthusiastic.

He was slender and he was bulky.

He was a recovering Catholic

He was a cultural Jew.

He was calm, thoughtful, and orderly.

He was animated, impulsive, and random.

Often he described him as a "stick,"

Meaning hard, formed, and inflexible.

In turn, he described him as a "sponge,"

Meaning soft, malleable, absorbing.

Over time the stick became more sponge-like.

The sponge became more stick-like.

Now one was becoming less

And one was having to become more.

Slowly while one was becoming the back partner

While one was becoming the front partner,

In this ménage à trois,

Alzheimer's was becoming the dominant partner.

*I include this poem here again many years later as it was one
which received many favorable reactions from readers.*

* * *

Epilogue – 11/18/15

It took Gregory four days to prepare to die.

It came on unexpectedly and quickly.

Hospice expected him to leave that day.

He slowed it down, allowing me time to process.

He was in no pain, his breathing not labored.

He was unresponsive, but knew I was there.

Knew I was talking to him and loving him,

I touched, stroked, petted him during the day.

Nurses kept a close eye on him overnight

I did not feel the need to keep a vigil.

He needed time to himself to prepare.

Compassionate, for others an even for himself.

On the third day of his coma,

He rallied his energy, gave me one last kiss.

He left his body calmly, a reflection of his life.

I celebrate him, I grieve him.

I continue to love him

✳ ✳ ✳

Normalcy Violated - 01/10/19

I worked so hard to keep our life normal.

Then something happens showing me

And to remind me that it is not normal.

That Dementia rules. And I react. Freak out.

Act in ways for which I know better.

I mistreated you because I love you so.

I lash out. I rage. I rage and lash out verbally.

I last out. I rage. I rage and last out physically.

Because I want our life to be normal, but it is not.

I want you to be safe, our life to be normal.

You are frightened, confused, frustrated.

So I lash out. I hit you. I slap you. I punish you.

Then I apologize. I cry. You cry. And I love you.

When normalcy disappears, I freak out. Lash out

I love you but it is not enough to just love you.

It should be enough, but it isn't enough.

I lash out and I freak out

And I apologize.

And I am so sorry.

And I cry.

And you cry.

And we love each other.

That should be enough

But sometimes it is not enough

And I lash out.

When will I learn?

Maybe next time.

Maybe next time?

Maybe ...

Next time.

On our anniversary, I revisited the difficult times while Gregory was still alive. I have forgiven myself knowing I am only human, was quick to apologize. If I could have, I would have been better. Gregory once said, "I do not expect you to change completely, just be here with me!"

✳ ✳ ✳

POETRY
WHILE OFF THE
ALZHEIMER'S
PATH

✳ ✳ ✳

SECTION THREE

<u>A Nun Goes Shopping - 07/20/19</u>

I laughed and I wondered.
She looks too old fashioned
to be ogling those red leather high heels
in the department store window.

He looks too old fashioned to be looking also
while left handedly fondling the nun's behind.
How did they get together, are they a couple,
do they even know each other.

Is she a nun and he the priest at the church,
together with all these years of celibacy?
He shows no emotion and neither does she
or maybe it just doesn't register with them.

Why would someone looking like him,
Balding and old and ugly be cupping a religious
Catholic nun's butt so thin and flabby and bony
somewhere under her black wool robes

✳ ✳ ✳

Poetry Distills Life - 07/30/19

Poetry distills life into its essence,

As we come upon four years.

Since my dear Gregory left

I miss him more than ever.

The writing does not come as often,

Nor as expressive, articulate, or eloquent,

With fewer emotional roller coaster rides,

Taken unexpectedly with him or now without.

I continue to grow and change and expand

While he does not, except in my memories.

So it seems to get easier, but in reality,

It never will be OK or be gone.

The circle of my life grows larger

New experiences, places, and people.

The circle of his death seemingly smaller

Remains as powerful as before, as ever.

I miss his touch, his smile, his smell,

I miss living my day to day with him,

My ups and downs, his shifts as well.

Someone with whom to share difficult times.

Laughter peeks it head out now and then,

But nowhere as much as it used to.

When joy gathers me in its arms

I am overwhelmed at the rare feeling.

The Roller Coaster ride has changed

But there are still ups and downs to weather.

So Gregory, Rest In Eternal Peace and

Michael, do your best to Live In Temporal Peace.

✳ ✳ ✳

<u>Doors – 08/25/19</u>

Doors will open wide, Doors will also close
Doors for which I will continue to be thankful
As they connect me with these caring others.

Those for whom I am so very grateful
For time spent working, playing, and learning
Some friendships which continue to this day.

They've helped me fill my days and weeks
With joyful adventure and serious times
With meaning in life which to me still speaks.

Change is good, but change has its own mind
I wish them well and do the same for myself
With love and emotions but with awareness.

That nothing is permanent
Everything changes
Whether you want it to or not!

* * *

Noisy Quiet & Chaotic Stillness - 03/30/21

COVID 19 has brought so many changes on us so quietly
    and so quickly.

People around the world are infected, either getting better
    or dying.

The harbingers of this change are invisible to the eye and
    all senses.

So we can only imagine what the black-hooded creature
    looks like.

Restaurants, museums, stores, schools, churches, libraries
    all close.

Events, conferences, music venues, plays, celebrations all
    turn off their lights.

Directly or indirectly; salaries, benefits, basic necessities
    are lost by many.

Those who have been suffering before are suffering even
    more now.

Outside and in, the quiet seems to feel so much more quiet
than before.
The stillness seems more still than usual and cities and
streets are empty.
The noise around us is so quiet that it deafens us in the
hearing of its roar.
And the darkness so great that it frightens each of us to
look at its approach.

We have come to expect that things will always be and
stay the same.
We expect that nothing will change or be rearranged in
our lives.
But in one day, all is different and unrecognizable and
incomprehensible.
And change is upon us, want it, like it, or not - we never
expected this.

Buddhist studies say that we should accept that all around
us is impermanent.
Knowing that every day everything around, in front and
behind us changes.
Even if imperceptible to the eye or ear or nose or taste or
sense of feeling.
Even if changes go unwanted or unnoticed, celebrated or
lamented.

From the time you woke up early very early this morning
on a Monday.
Everything about your physical being is no longer the
same later on a Tuesday.
Cells have died off, sluffed off, been rearranged or
renewed by Wednesday.
Organs do their job pumping, breathing, breaking down
components on Thursday.

What might be the same, you think, is your attitude and
  your belief system.
You might think the same thoughts you have always had
  about things and life around.
Your actions and reactions follow the same triggers that
  you have used before.
But suddenly they may no longer apply, be true, be
  appropriate, or be necessary.

So in this time of great change for all of in the world,
  young and old.
If we can change with the times it could become easier to
  feel the air.
As we vow to change our antiquated thoughts and actions
  and triggers.
We build a new you to reflect who you have or will
  become with new attitudes.

Have faith in yourself to know that it is OK where you are
    at and that you will grow.
Have faith in your fellow humans that we will survive this
    and come out the other side.
We will experience change and seek out the good in
    change and become stronger.
And the world will most likely be a better place for all,
    because it certainly needs to be.

The quiet seems more beautiful to hear, the stillness seems
    more beautiful to experience.
The noise seems so quiet that we can hear the birds make
    their music, sing their songs.
The fear so great it energizes one to step up to change and
    recognize the gift that we have.
And we will continue to tell our stories of hope, and love,
    and compassion, and life

THE EVERYTHING POEM

By: Tukaram

I am looking for a poem that says
Everything so I don't have to write anymore.

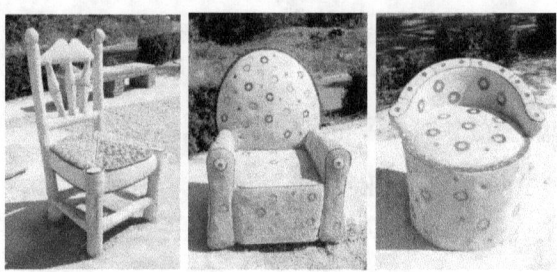

Ending this Volume 3 of Poetry with a poem by Tukaram 1608-1649. His genius partly lies in his ability to transform the external world into its spiritual analogue.

Tukaram's stature in Marathi literature is comparable to that of Shakespeare in English. He could be called the quintessential Marathi poet reflecting the genius or the language as well as its characteristic literary culture.

COME SIT WITH ME
ANOTHER WHILE LONGER
CHAIR PHOTOGRAPHS

SECTION FOUR

These photographs, taken by Michael, are located in the Evanston condo, home to Gregory (RIP October 4, 2015) and Michael and cats Emma and Gigi.

Join me and SIT ANOTHER WHILE LONGER as we contemplate life and our place in it. NAMASTE!

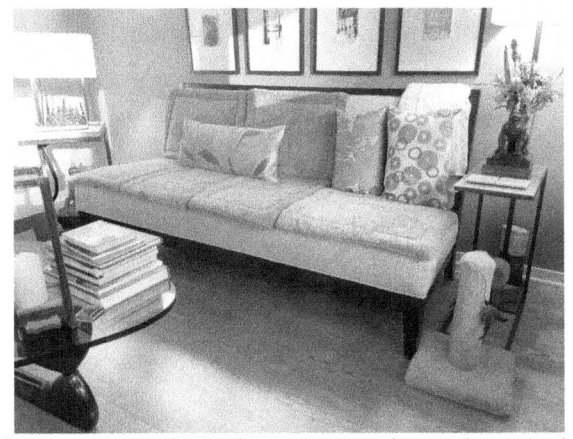

Not really a chair, but we can sit on the couch
and talk about love and other things.

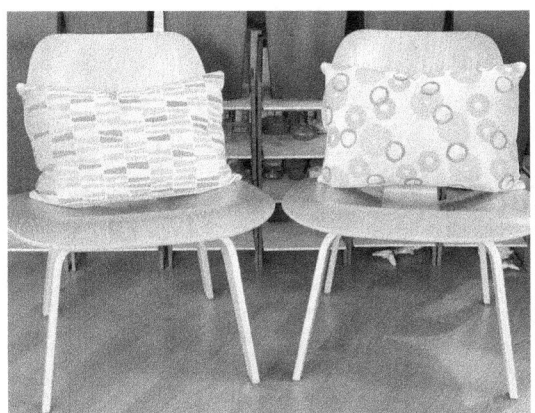

Livingroom chairs, comfy place to sit
and chat or watch the sun rise.

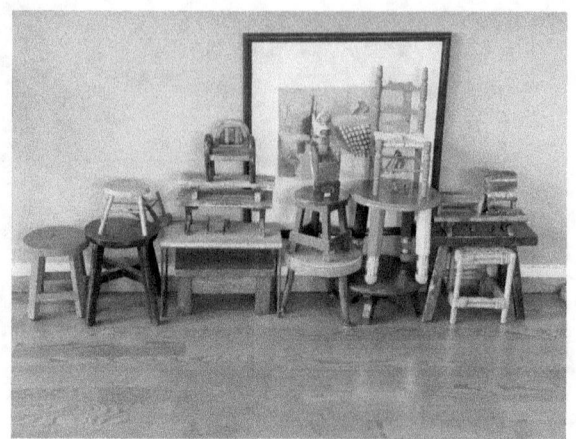

Collection of miniature chairs and stools.
Many were gifts from family and friends.

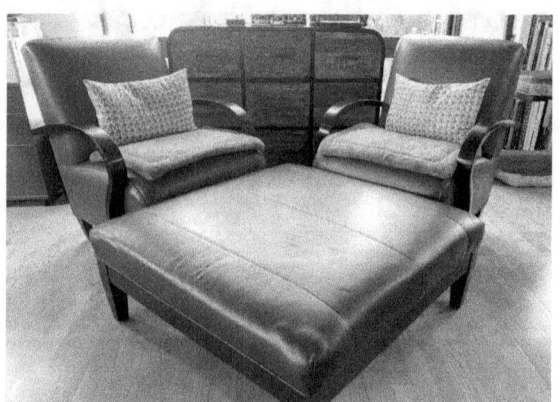

Livingroom chairs and ottoman.
Put your feet up and let's talk about life.

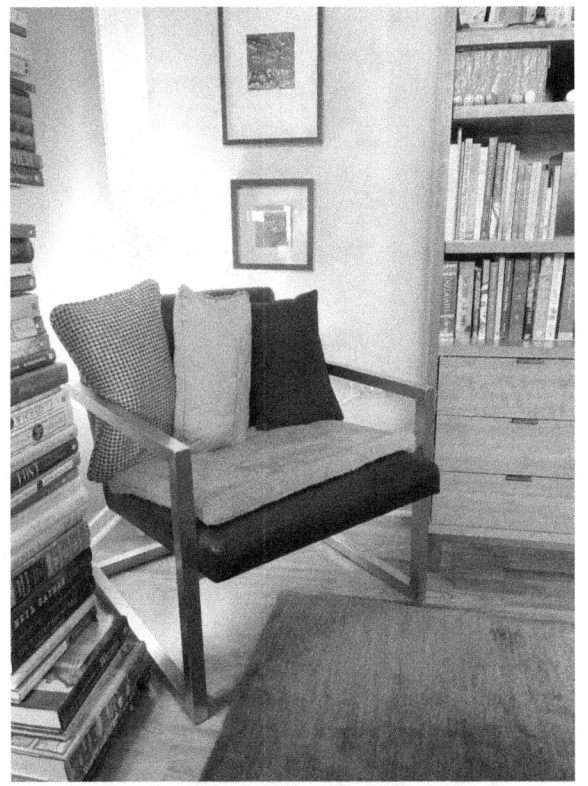

Michael's reading corner chair in master bedroom.
Great with a new book of poetry to read.

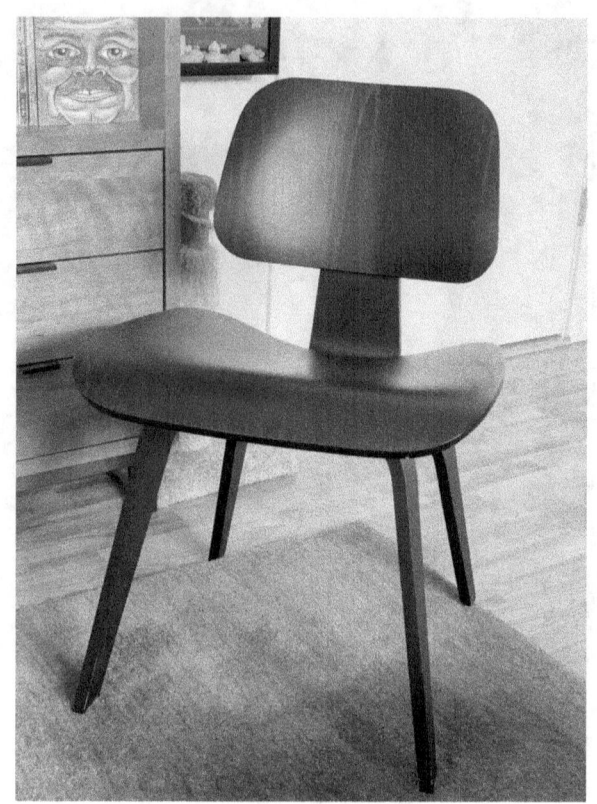

Guest's reading corner chair in master bedroom.
Grab a book and let's read together.

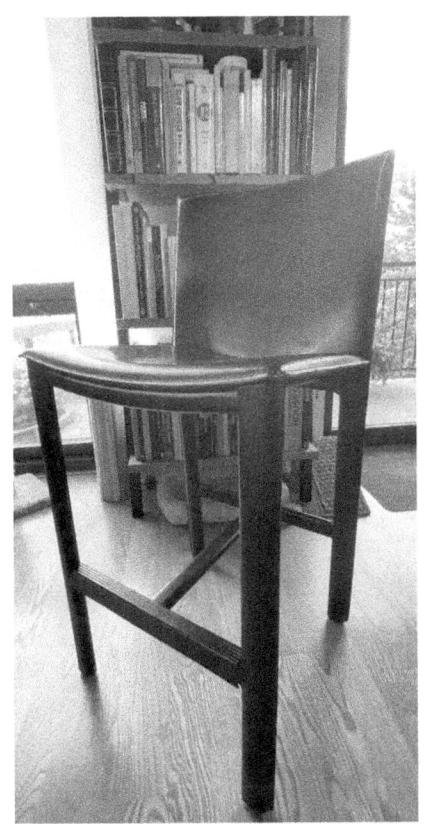

A stool at the kitchen counter, where meals take
place, or we can just have a cup of coffee
and some freshly baked chocolate chip cookies.

INDICES

ABOUT MICHAEL

Michael Horvich is a retired educator, administrator, and college instructor. He is currently a writer, artist, collector, museum curator, photographer, jewelry artist, and actor. He has won two Fellowships in Gifted Education from the State of Illinois, a Performing Arts Grant from the City of Chicago, and a residency in non-fiction writing with The Ragdale Foundation in Lake Forest, Illinois. Michael has been published in a number of educational journals. He has appeared on stage as a Supernumerary at the Lyric Opera of Chicago in over twenty operas. Michael's Museum, a collection of over 105 collections of Tiny Treasures was installed as a permanent exhibit at The Chicago Children's Museum on Navy Pier in May 2011. He is currently working on his memoirs: "GYROSCOPE: An Alzheimer's Love Story. He lives in Evanston, Illinois with his life partner Gregory and their cat Mariah.

FOLLOW MICHAEL

Site: www.horvich.com

E-Mail: m@horvich.com

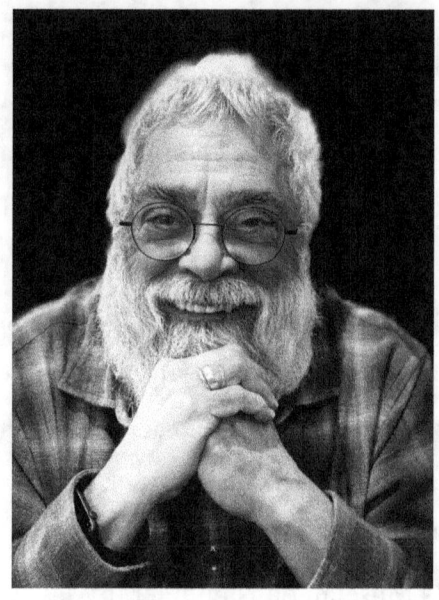

BOOKS BY MICHAEL

AVAILABLE AT
www.amazon.com, www.barnesandnoble.com
www.lulu.com

SIT WITH ME A WHILE
The Collected Works of Michael A. Horvich
2000-2010

SIT WITH ME A WHILE LONGER
The Collected Works of Michael A. Horvich
2011-2013

THE STORY OF
MICHAEL'S MUSEUM:
A Curious Collection of Tiny Treasures
*(Now a permanent exhibit at Chicago Children's Museum
Navy Pier, Chicago, Illinois)*

COUNTING DOWN THE
YARDSTICK:
A Reincarnation Memoir

MUSEUM OF MICHAEL'S MIND:
Memories, Memoirs, and Meanderings Volume 1

MUSEUM OF MICHAEL'S MIND:
Memories, Memoirs, and Meanderings Volume II

GYROSCOPE:
An Alzheimer's Love Story
The Joys, The Sorrows, and The Gifts of Dementia

A PONDERING
Thoughts on Thinking

POETRY

Sit With Me A While Longer

The Collected Works
of Michael A. Horvich
2011-2013
and a few earlier ones

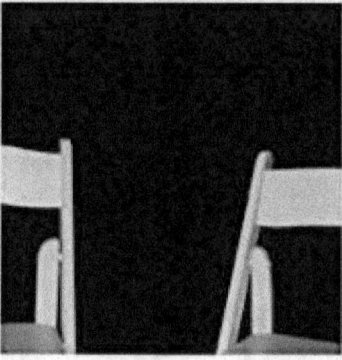

POETRY

Sit With Me A While

The Collected Works
of Michael A. Horvich
2000 - 2010

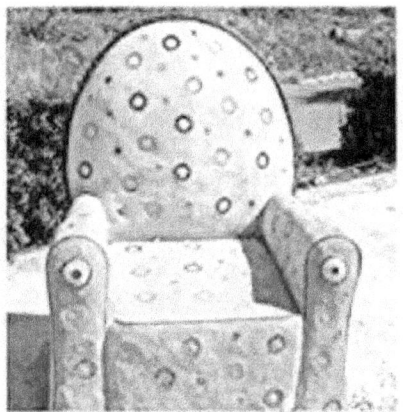

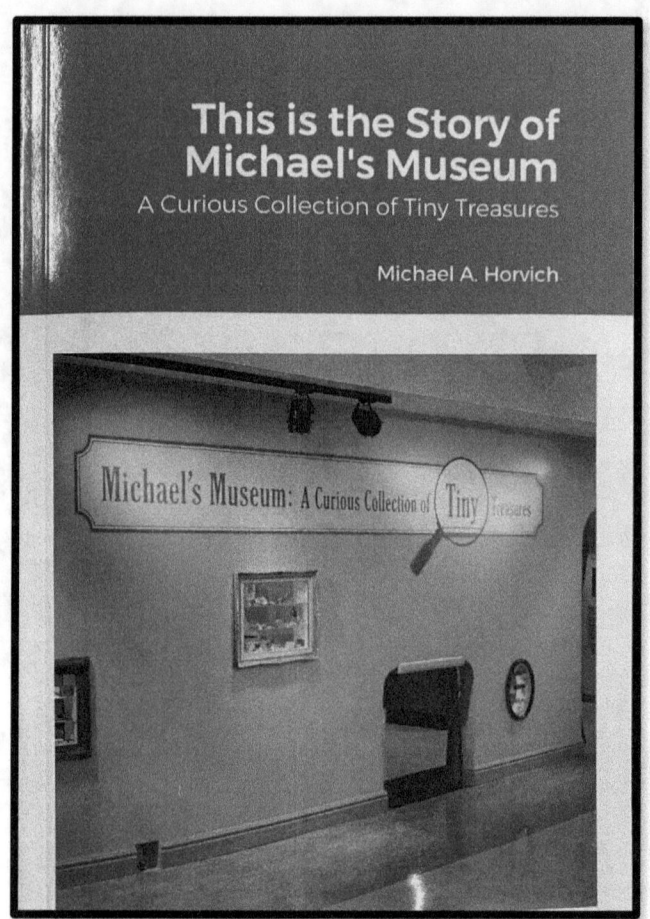

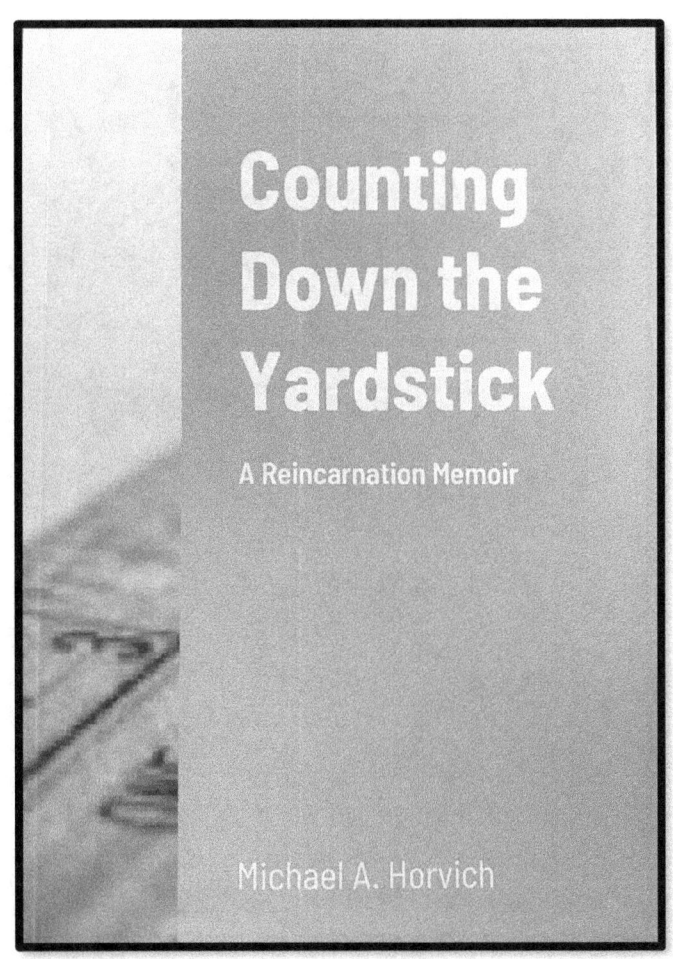

Counting Down the Yardstick

A Reincarnation Memoir

Michael A. Horvich

The Museum of Michael's
Mind: Memories, Memoirs,
and Meanderings

Volume One: The Collected Writings
2005—2015

By: Michael A. Horvich

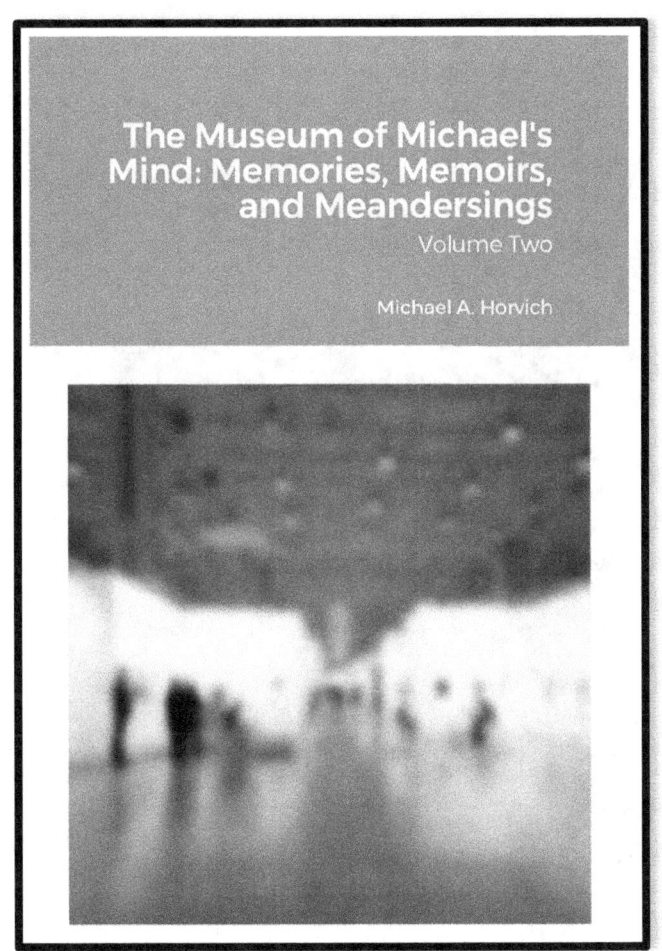

The Museum of Michael's
Mind: Memories, Memoirs,
and Meandersings
Volume Two

Michael A. Horvich

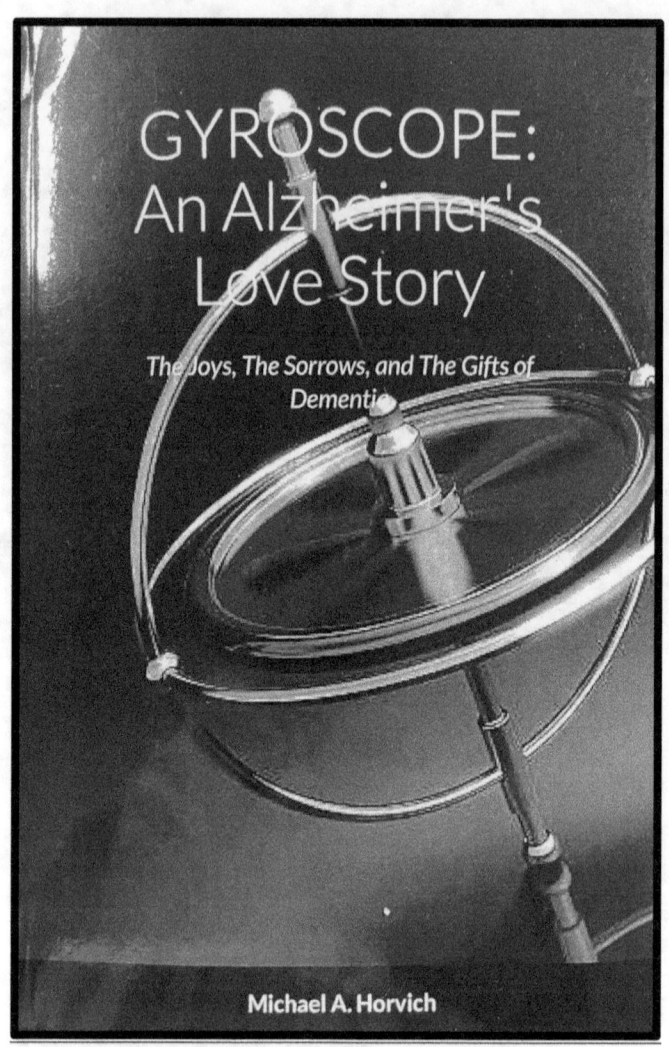

GYROSCOPE:
An Alzheimer's
Love Story

The Joys, The Sorrows, and The Gifts of
Dementia

Michael A. Horvich

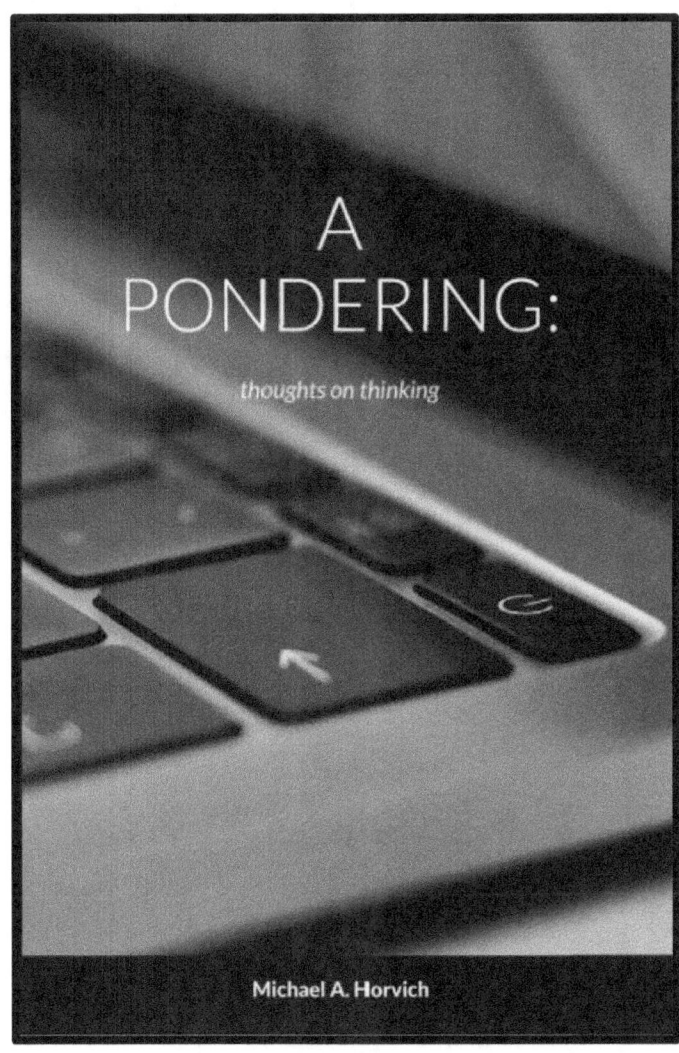

A
PONDERING:

thoughts on thinking

Michael A. Horvich

www.ingramcontent.com/pod-product-compliance
Lightning Source LLC
Chambersburg PA
CBHW070306290526
45791CB00003B/1096